Medicinal Mushrooms

A Beginner's 5-Step Quick Start Guide on Getting Started, with an Overview of its Health Use Cases

FELICITY PAULMAN

Disclaimer

By reading this disclaimer, you are accepting the terms of the disclaimer in full. If you disagree with this disclaimer, please do not read the guide.

All of the content within this guide is provided for informational and educational purposes only, and should not be accepted as independent medical or other professional advice. The author is not a doctor, physician, nurse, mental health provider, or registered nutritionist/dietician. Therefore, using and reading this guide does not establish any form of a physician-patient relationship.

Always consult with a physician or another qualified health provider with any issues or questions you might have regarding any sort of medical condition. Do not ever disregard any qualified professional medical advice or delay seeking that advice because of anything you have read in this guide. The information in this guide is not intended to be any sort of medical advice and should not be used in lieu of any medical advice by a licensed and qualified medical professional.

The information in this guide has been compiled from a variety of known sources. However, the author cannot attest to or guarantee the accuracy of each source and thus should not be held liable for any errors or omissions.

Introduction

Are you looking for a natural and effective way to improve your overall health and well-being? Have you heard about the incredible benefits of medicinal mushrooms? If you're interested in exploring the world of natural remedies, medicinal mushrooms may be just what you're looking for.

Medicinal mushrooms have been used for centuries in traditional medicine practices around the world. From China to Europe to North America, these powerful fungi have been recognized for their healing properties and are now gaining popularity in Western medicine as well. With over 14,000 species of mushrooms, there is a vast array of options to choose from, each with its unique set of benefits.

In this guide, we will explore the following;

- What is a Medicinal Mushroom?
- Different Types of Medicinal Mushrooms
- Preparation Methods
- Side Effects
- Benefits of Medicinal Mushrooms
- Advantages and Disadvantages of Medicinal Mushrooms
- Bioactive Compounds Found in Medicinal Mushrooms
- Use Cases

- 5-Step Guide to Getting Started the Medicinal Mushrooms
- Safety Considerations

With so many options to choose from, it can be overwhelming to know where to start when incorporating medicinal mushrooms into your daily routine. By the end of this guide, you will have a better understanding of which mushrooms are best suited to your individual needs and how to use them to support your health goals.

Don't miss out on the opportunity to enhance your health through the power of medicinal mushrooms. Keep reading to discover the incredible benefits they have to offer, and take the first step towards a healthier, happier you.

Table of Contents

CHAPTER 1: WHAT IS MEDICINAL MUSHROOM?

Medicinal mushrooms are fungi that have been used for centuries in traditional medicine systems around the world. These mushrooms contain a range of bioactive compounds, including polysaccharides, triterpenoids, and sterols, which have been shown to have various health benefits such as boosting immune function, reducing inflammation, and promoting digestive health.

However, it is important to consider safety considerations when consuming medicinal mushrooms. Some types of medicinal mushrooms can interact with certain medical conditions or other supplements and herbs. Additionally, improper preparation or storage of medicinal mushrooms can lead to contamination or spoilage, causing adverse reactions.

To ensure the safety and effectiveness of medicinal mushroom consumption, it is important to consult with a healthcare provider before starting any new supplement regimen. It is also important to follow proper dosage guidelines and purchase high-quality mushrooms from reputable sources.

In the next section, we will delve more into different types of mushrooms and some preparation methods. So keep reading to learn more.

Different Types of Medicinal Mushrooms

There are a wide variety of medicinal mushrooms available, each containing its own unique set of active compounds. Here is an overview of some popular varieties and their purported health benefits:

- **Reishi:** A popular mushroom in Traditional Chinese Medicine, Reishi is known for its immune-boosting properties. It contains beta-glucans, which help stimulate the immune system and may even have anti-cancer effects.
- **Lion's Mane:** Named for its shaggy white appearance, Lion's Mane is considered a nootropic mushroom due to its ability to enhance cognitive function. It contains compounds called hericenones and erinacines, which may stimulate nerve growth and protect against neurological diseases.
- **Chaga:** Found primarily on birch trees in cold climates, Chaga has been used for centuries in Russia and Scandinavia as a folk remedy. It's rich in antioxidants and may have anti-inflammatory effects, making it potentially helpful for various health conditions.
- **Cordyceps:** Grown on the larvae of insects, Cordyceps is often used for its energy-boosting properties. It can increase oxygen uptake in the body,

improve athletic performance, and may even have anti-aging effects.

- **Turkey Tail:** This colorful mushroom is often used in traditional medicine to support the immune system. It contains polysaccharides that may help stimulate the immune system and has been studied for its potential anti-cancer effects.

- **Maitake:** Also known as "Hen of the Woods," Maitake is a popular edible mushroom that also has medicinal properties. It contains beta-glucans that may help boost the immune system and may also have hypoglycemic effects, making it potentially helpful for those with diabetes.

- **Shiitake:** Often used in cooking, Shiitake is also considered a medicinal mushroom. It contains a compound called lentinan, which has been shown to stimulate the immune system and has been studied for its potential anti-cancer effects.

- **Tremella:** also known as "snow fungus," is a jelly-like mushroom that has been used in traditional Chinese medicine for thousands of years. It's rich in antioxidants and may help boost collagen production, making it potentially beneficial for skin health

- **Agaricus blazei:** Originating in Brazil, Agaricus blazei is a potent immune booster that's been shown to have anti-tumor properties. It contains beta-glucans and other polysaccharides that stimulate the immune system and may help reduce inflammation.

- **Poria:** Poria is a woody mushroom that's been used for centuries in traditional Chinese medicine to support the immune system and promote digestive health. It contains triterpenes, which have been shown to have anti-inflammatory effects.

- **Phellinus linteus:** Also known as "Mishima" in Japan, Phellinus linteus is a potent anti-cancer mushroom that's been used in traditional medicine for centuries. It contains compounds called ergosterols, which have been shown to inhibit the growth of cancer cells.

- **Agarikon:** Agarikon is a rare mushroom that grows primarily in old-growth forests of the Pacific Northwest. It's been used for centuries by indigenous people for its immune-boosting properties and may have antiviral effects.

- **Enoki:** A popular culinary mushroom in Asian cuisine, Enoki also has medicinal properties. It contains antioxidants and may have anti-inflammatory effects, making it potentially helpful for various health conditions.

These are just a few of the many species of medicinal mushrooms available. Many more have yet to be studied, so it's important to do your research before adding any new supplement to your health regimen.

Preparation Methods

Medicinal mushrooms can be consumed in several different ways, including fresh or dried, as a tea, tincture, or supplement. Here are some common methods of preparing medicinal mushrooms:

Decoction

The preparation of therapeutic mushrooms frequently involves the use of a decoction. To extract the beneficial chemicals from dried mushroom pieces, this method entails boiling the pieces in water for an extended period. The use of decoction is one of the most efficient methods for extracting the medicinal benefits of mushrooms because it enables a more concentrated and powerful extraction of the mushrooms' active components.

Because of its beneficial effects on one's health, the liquid that is produced can either be used to make tea or added to other foods and beverages. Individuals may simply incorporate these nutrient-dense mushrooms into their daily routine by adopting this technique of preparation, and in doing so, take advantage of the myriad of health benefits that these mushrooms have to offer.

Powdered extracts

The adaptability and portability of powdered medicinal mushroom extracts have contributed to their meteoric rise in popularity in recent years. These extracts are produced by drying and grinding the mushrooms into a fine powder, which can then be readily added to a range of other recipes. The mushrooms are first dried and then ground into powder. Smoothies, soups, and other types of foods, in addition to providing a variety of health benefits, can benefit from the use of medicinal mushroom powders.

Depending on the type of mushroom that was used to make the powder, its potential health benefits may include enhancing cognitive function, boosting the immune system, reducing inflammation, or supporting overall wellness. They make it easy and convenient to reap the benefits of medicinal mushrooms as part of one's routine, and they are very efficient at doing so.

Tinctures

Tinctures made from medicinal mushrooms are a common method for obtaining therapeutic components extracted from a variety of mushrooms. The mushrooms are extracted from their active compounds through a process that involves soaking them in alcohol or another solvent. After that, these tinctures are diluted with water or other liquids and taken orally in very small doses to benefit from their medical effects.

Tinctures are not the only technique to extract these helpful components; however, they are a method that is practical, efficient, and may be easily incorporated into one's daily routine. In addition, tinctures make it possible to extract these useful components more effectively and efficiently, which results in a final product that is both more potent and more useful.

Capsules

Consuming medicinal mushrooms through the use of capsules is quickly becoming one of the most common and practical options available. The mushroom extracts included within the capsules have been finely pulverized, making them simple to swallow. Additionally, the capsules contain a higher concentration of active chemicals compared to other types of mushroom supplements, such as powders or teas.

Furthermore, capsules are easier to transport and have a longer shelf life, making them a suitable option for individuals who want to incorporate the health advantages of medicinal mushrooms into their daily routines but are unsure how to do so. Reishi, Chaga, Lion's Mane, and Cordyceps are some of the mushroom species that are most frequently consumed in capsule form.

Raw

The eating of raw medicinal mushrooms, particularly shiitake and maitake kinds, is garnering an ever-increasing amount of attention and interest. Some of the chemicals and minerals found in these mushrooms, such as beta-glucans and polysaccharides, have been shown to have a positive impact on human health.

When adding raw mushrooms to dishes or salads, it is necessary to make sure the mushrooms are well-washed and sliced very thinly so that they are easier to digest. Raw mushrooms are an interesting and potentially nutritious addition to anyone's diet; however, some people prefer to prepare their mushrooms to eliminate any potential toxins. If cooked properly, mushrooms can be consumed safely.

Cooking

Cooking medicinal mushrooms by sautéing, roasting, or grilling them is an excellent approach to preparing them. The mushrooms are fried in a skillet with butter or oil, and the cooking process is continued until the mushrooms are soft. Roasting is a method that uses dry heat and involves placing the mushrooms in an oven. The heat from the oven causes the mushrooms to become caramelized and crispy.

The taste of the mushrooms is enhanced by the grilling process, which imparts a smokey flavor and gives them more dimension. These preparation methods not only improve the taste, but also preserve vital nutrients such as beta-glucans and polysaccharides, both of which are good for the body and contribute to overall wellness.

Fermented

Fermenting medicinal mushrooms is a one-of-a-kind and highly effective method for taking advantage of the health advantages offered by these mushrooms. Through the process of fermentation, the complex compounds that are contained in mushrooms are broken down, which both increases the bioavailability of the mushrooms and makes it easier for the body to absorb them.

The use of fermented mushroom products like kombucha and kimchi, which both contain helpful bacteria and enzymes, can assist in improving general gut health. These products can be a wonderful addition to any diet because they offer a savory and simple method for ingesting medicinal mushrooms that is also gentle on the digestive system.

Topical use

The preparation of skin creams or ointments made from various extracts of medicinal mushrooms is known as the topical usage of medicinal mushrooms. It is claimed that these products offer a variety of benefits to the skin, such as enhancing the skin's ability to retain moisture, fostering the production of collagen, and alleviating inflammation. Reishi, cordyceps, and chaga are just a few examples of therapeutic mushrooms that are frequently applied topically, along with a plethora of other varieties.

The effectiveness of these preparations may vary depending on the type of mushroom, its concentration, and the specific condition being treated. However, many people find relief and improvement in their skin health by using topical mushroom preparations.

Regardless of the preparation method, it's important to purchase high-quality medicinal mushrooms from reputable sources and to follow dosage instructions carefully to ensure safe and effective use.

Bioactive Compounds Found in Mushrooms

In addition to the numerous potential health benefits of medicinal mushrooms, it is important to understand the bioactive compounds that are found in these fungi. Bioactive compounds are substances within the mushroom that interact with cells and may affect different processes in the body. These compounds include;

Beta-glucans

Beta-glucans are complex polysaccharides found in various medicinal mushroom species like shiitake, maitake, and reishi. The immune system-stimulating properties of beta-glucans make them a potent bioactive compound for preventing chronic diseases and fighting infections.

Beta-glucans modulate the immune system's response by positively influencing immune cells, ultimately promoting their optimal function. Nevertheless, the crucial fact is, each mushroom species contains distinct beta-glucans chemical structures that possess different functionalities and immune-boosting potential.

Triterpenoids

Triterpenoids are a group of bioactive compounds found in medicinal mushrooms, particularly in reishi mushrooms. These compounds have been extensively studied for their anti-inflammatory, antioxidant, and anticancer properties. Research has shown that triterpenoids may also support liver function by reducing inflammation and oxidative stress.

Moreover, they have been found to have anti-anxiety and anti-depressive effects, making them a potential natural remedy for stress-related disorders. Triterpenoids are believed to work by modulating various signaling pathways in the body, including the immune, oxidative, and neuroendocrine systems. Their synergistic effects with other bioactive compounds in medicinal mushrooms make them a promising target for drug development and nutraceutical production.

Polysaccharides

Polysaccharides are a class of bioactive compounds found in certain medicinal mushrooms, such as shiitake, maitake, cordyceps, and lion's mane. These long-chain carbohydrates have been found to possess antioxidant, anti-inflammatory, and immune-stimulating properties, among others.

Studies have suggested that polysaccharides may be beneficial for various health conditions, including cancer, cardiovascular disease, and autoimmune disorders. They may also support cognitive function and help regulate blood sugar levels. Overall, polysaccharides demonstrate the potential for medicinal mushrooms as promising natural remedies with multiple health benefits.

Ergosterol

Ergosterol is a bioactive compound found in certain species of medicinal mushrooms like shiitake and maitake. It is a precursor to vitamin D, which plays a vital role in supporting bone health and immune function. When ergosterol is exposed to UV light, it is converted into vitamin D2 known to reduce the risk of osteoporosis and bone fractures.

Additionally, ergosterol promotes the body's natural defense mechanisms against harmful threats, strengthening the immune system. Hence, medicinal mushrooms are a potential source of ergosterol, providing several health benefits for optimum wellness.

Polyphenols

Polyphenols are potent antioxidant compounds that can be found abundantly in several types of medicinal mushrooms like Chaga and reishi. These bioactive compounds hold a significant role in protecting against oxidative stress and damage caused by free radicals in the human body.

Recent research suggests that polyphenols may also exhibit anti-inflammatory and anti-cancer properties, making them a promising ingredient in various health and wellness products. Despite the numerous health benefits that polyphenols offer, sufficient scientific evidence is still needed to explore and validate their full potential in treating and preventing various diseases.

Adenosine

Adenosine, a nucleoside found in medicinal mushrooms like cordyceps, has been found to possess several health benefits. It has been shown to exhibit anti-inflammatory and anti-platelet properties, which contribute to its potential in supporting cardiovascular and respiratory function.

Additionally, adenosine may play a role in regulating immune system function and promoting healthy aging. Further research is needed to fully understand the extent of adenosine's therapeutic properties, but its presence in medicinal mushrooms highlights the importance of these natural sources in promoting overall health and wellness.

Overall, the bioactive compounds found in medicinal mushrooms are numerous and varied, and each species of mushroom contains a unique combination of these compounds. By understanding the bioactive compounds in medicinal mushrooms, it is possible to choose the right mushroom for your specific health needs and goals.

Side Effects

While medicinal mushrooms are generally considered safe for most people, they may cause side effects in some individuals. Here are some potential side effects of using medicinal mushrooms:

- **Allergic reactions:** Some people may be allergic to certain types of mushrooms, which can cause symptoms such as itching, rash, and difficulty breathing.
- **Gastrointestinal upset:** In some cases, consuming too many medicinal mushrooms or using them in the wrong form can cause digestive discomfort such as gas, bloating, and diarrhea.
- **Blood sugar changes:** Some medicinal mushrooms may have an impact on blood sugar levels, which can be problematic for individuals with diabetes or other blood sugar disorders.
- **Interaction with medications:** Some medicinal mushrooms may interact with certain medications, including blood thinners and immunosuppressants.
- **Vitamin D toxicity:** Certain medicinal mushrooms are high in vitamin D, and taking too many of these mushrooms or supplements can lead to vitamin D toxicity.
- **Headaches:** In some cases, consuming certain medicinal mushrooms or supplements may cause headaches.

- **Nausea:** Some people may experience nausea or vomiting after consuming medicinal mushrooms, especially in large quantities.
- **Skin reactions:** In rare cases, topical use of medicinal mushrooms (such as in creams or ointments) may cause skin irritation, rashes, or other allergic reactions.
- **Lowered blood pressure:** Some mushroom species have been found to have blood pressure-lowering effects, which can be problematic for individuals with already low blood pressure.
- **Liver toxicity:** Certain mushroom species contain compounds that can be toxic to the liver if consumed in large quantities.

It's important to remember that these side effects are relatively uncommon, and most people can use medicinal mushrooms safely and without any adverse effects. However, it's always a good idea to consult with a healthcare professional before starting to use medicinal mushrooms to ensure they're safe for you to use and won't interfere with any other medications or treatments you may be taking.

CHAPTER 2: BENEFITS OF MEDICINAL MUSHROOMS

Medicinal mushrooms are gaining popularity as more people recognize their potential health benefits. These amazing fungi contain a wealth of compounds that have been found to have anti-inflammatory, immune-boosting, and even anti-cancer effects. However, like any supplement or medication, medicinal mushrooms may also come with potential disadvantages.

In this chapter, we'll explore the potential benefits of medicinal mushrooms, as well as some of the disadvantages you should be aware of. Whether you're a seasoned mushroom enthusiast or just starting to explore their potential, this guide will provide you with the information you need to make informed decisions about your health.

Benefits of Medicinal Mushrooms

Medicinal mushrooms have been used for centuries in traditional medicine to treat a wide range of health conditions. Here are some of the potential benefits of using medicinal mushrooms:

Immune system support

The use of medicinal mushrooms has been shown to have significant benefits for the maintenance of the immune system. Compounds that can be found in mushrooms, such as beta-glucans and polysaccharides, have been proven to boost immune cell activity, increase antibody production, and possibly even have anti-tumor effects. These benefits can be attributed to the mushrooms' beta-glucans and polysaccharides.

People who suffer from autoimmune illnesses, allergies, or other conditions related to the immune system may benefit significantly from these effects. In addition, medicinal mushrooms may also give benefits related to antioxidants and anti-inflammatory properties, which makes them a potentially useful adjunct therapy for the health of the immune system.

Moreover, studies have shown that certain mushroom extracts may have immunomodulatory properties that can support cancer treatment. With these potential benefits, medicinal mushrooms offer a fascinating avenue for future research and therapeutic development in immune system intervention.

Anti-inflammatory effects

It has been discovered that specific constituent components of medicinal mushrooms have anti-inflammatory effects, and these benefits have been the subject of research. These substances have the potential to assist in the relief of symptoms associated with inflammatory disorders, such as allergies and arthritis.

According to the findings of one study, the lion's mane mushroom can lessen the inflammation and pain caused by nerve injury. According to the findings of yet another study, reishi mushrooms have the potential to reduce inflammation in the airways of asthma patients. According to these findings, utilizing medicinal mushrooms as part of a treatment plan may provide a viable alternative to the use of conventional anti-inflammatory medications.

Antioxidant effects

Because it has a high concentration of naturally occurring chemicals, the medicinal mushroom known as Cordyceps sinensis has been discovered to have powerful antioxidant capabilities. Free radicals, which can be harmful to DNA and lead to a variety of diseases, are neutralized by these antioxidants, which in turn protect the cells of the body from harm.

Ergothioneine, which may be found in cordyceps, is known for its powerful antioxidant properties and is one of the components of cordyceps. Because of this, cordyceps has a lot of potential as a natural medicine that can help support general health and wellness.

Cholesterol-lowering effects

It has been shown that medicinal mushrooms provide a variety of benefits to one's health, including the possibility of lowering one's cholesterol levels and reducing the chance of developing cardiovascular disease. According to research, particular kinds of mushroom extracts may be able to assist inhibit the absorption of cholesterol in the stomach, which would lead to a decrease in overall cholesterol levels.

Compounds found in mushrooms, such as beta-glucans and ergothioneine, have also been linked to improved heart health. Incorporating medicinal mushrooms into a balanced and healthy diet may be a natural and effective way to support cardiovascular health.

Blood sugar regulation

Medicinal mushrooms are an excellent natural option to regulate blood sugar levels due to their anti-diabetic effects. They contain bioactive compounds such as polysaccharides and beta-glucans, which have been found to improve insulin sensitivity and glucose metabolism.

The polysaccharides present in mushrooms act as an insulin mimetic, binding to the insulin receptors and promoting glucose uptake by the cells. Additionally, the beta-glucans found in mushrooms prevent the absorption of glucose in the intestines, leading to lower blood sugar levels.

This is particularly beneficial for people with type 2 diabetes, as it helps to improve glycemic control and reduce the risk of complications associated with high blood sugar levels.

Cognitive function improvement

It has been discovered that medicinal mushrooms contain chemicals that can improve cognitive function. These chemicals have neuroprotective characteristics, which help maintain healthy brain function and protect against harm to the brain.

Additionally, medicinal mushrooms have been shown to alleviate symptoms of anxiety and depression. Research has found that certain species of mushrooms, including Lion's Mane and Reishi, can improve memory, focus, and overall brain health. Incorporating medicinal mushrooms into one's diet or supplement routine may provide numerous cognitive benefits.

Adaptogenic effects

Medicinal mushroom species such as Reishi, Cordyceps, and Lion's Mane have adaptogenic compounds that can improve the body's response to stress and fatigue. These adaptogens activate the body's natural defense mechanisms, boost immunity, and help maintain homeostasis.

Studies have shown that regular consumption of these mushrooms can support better physical and mental health, improve athletic performance, and reduce the risk of chronic diseases associated with stress. Additionally, these mushrooms also possess antioxidant and anti-inflammatory properties that can further enhance their health benefits.

While more research is needed to fully understand the potential benefits of medicinal mushrooms, many people have reported positive effects from using them in combination with conventional treatments.

It's important to consult with a healthcare professional before starting to use medicinal mushrooms to ensure they're safe for you to use and won't interfere with any other medications or treatments you may be taking.

Advantages of Medicinal Mushrooms

In addition to the potential health benefits, medicinal mushrooms may also offer an array of advantages. For example, they are easy to find and relatively inexpensive compared to other supplements.

They often have fewer side effects than pharmaceutical drugs, making them a good alternative for those who prefer natural remedies.

Some of the advantages include the following;

Low maintenance

Growing medicinal mushrooms at home require very little in the way of equipment and upkeep, which makes them both an affordable and environmentally responsible alternative for a healthy diet. Growing oyster and shiitake mushrooms requires very little attention and care and can even be done in confined locations with only a little bit of room.

These mushrooms are excellent sources of antioxidants, vitamins, and minerals, including vitamin D and potassium. Incorporating these nutrient-rich fungi into a diet can benefit both physical health, such as immune system support, and decreased inflammation, and mental health, as they contain compounds that may boost mood and cognitive function.

Sustainable

Medicinal mushrooms provide a sustainable food source as they can be grown using agricultural byproducts or waste products. This method not only ensures the preservation of the environment but also contributes to reducing food waste. Moreover, medicinal mushrooms can be harvested from the wild, without causing harm to natural ecosystems.

This helps maintain the biodiversity of forests and supports the local economy. Growing mushrooms also require less land and water compared to livestock farming, making it an eco-friendly alternative. Overall, medicinal mushrooms are a smart choice for individuals who prioritize sustainability and eco-friendliness.

Cost-effective

Medicinal mushrooms offer a cost-effective option for those seeking to improve their overall health. Compared to other supplements or medications, they are often more affordable and can be grown at home with ease. Furthermore, they are known to have a range of benefits, from boosting the immune system to reducing inflammation in the body.

As such, incorporating medicinal mushrooms into one's diet can be a wise investment in one's long-term well-being.

Versatile

One of the major advantages of medicinal mushrooms is their versatility. They can be used in a wide range of dishes, including soups, stews, risottos, and stir-fries, allowing people to enjoy their unique flavor and nutritional benefits in many different ways. Additionally, these mushrooms are available in a variety of forms, such as powders, capsules, and tinctures, making them easy and convenient to add to one's daily routine.

They are also popular for their immune-boosting properties, which have been attributed to their polysaccharides and other bioactive compounds. Overall, medicinal mushrooms offer a delicious and practical way to enhance both the taste and nutritional value of any meal, as well as provide a range of potential health benefits.

Culturally significant

The advantage of incorporating medicinal mushrooms into one's health routine is their cultural significance and historical use in traditional medicine systems. Many cultures from around the world have recognized their health benefits and have used them for centuries. For example, Reishi mushrooms have been used in traditional Chinese medicine to boost the immune system, reduce inflammation, and improve heart health.

Similarly, Chaga mushrooms have been used in Siberian traditional medicine to treat respiratory infections, lower blood pressure, and cholesterol levels, and improve digestion. Thus, opting for medicinal mushrooms in one's diet not only provides health benefits but also promotes cultural and historical practices.

Overall, medicinal mushrooms offer a range of advantages, including being low maintenance, sustainable, cost-effective, versatile, culturally significant, and potentially beneficial for health and wellness. Incorporating medicinal mushrooms into your diet or supplement regimen may provide a natural way to support your health and well-being.

Disadvantages of Medicinal Mushrooms

While medicinal mushrooms have many potential benefits, they may also come with some disadvantages. However, for most people, the benefits of medicinal mushrooms will outweigh any potential risks. Here are some of the disadvantages to keep in mind:

Possible allergic reactions

Those who are allergic to certain types of mushrooms may experience adverse reactions when consuming medicinal mushrooms, which is a notable disadvantage. Symptoms can range from mild to severe, including itching, swelling of the face or throat, difficulty breathing, and even anaphylaxis.

Individuals with known allergies to mushrooms must avoid the consumption of medicinal mushrooms or consult with a healthcare professional before doing so. However, for those who are not allergic, medicinal mushrooms offer a wide range of potential health benefits and should be considered as part of a balanced diet.

Potential interactions with medications

Medicinal mushrooms are known for their health benefits, but they can potentially interact with certain medications. For instance, blood thinners and immunosuppressants can be negatively affected when taken with medicinal mushrooms, as they can cause interactions that could lead to serious health issues. It is essential to consult a healthcare professional before adding medicinal mushrooms to one's diet to avoid any negative drug interactions.

Variability in quality

Consumers should be cautious when purchasing medicinal mushroom supplements due to the wide variability in quality and potency. The lack of regulation in the industry means that some brands may not contain as many of the active compounds as claimed on the label, while others may be contaminated with harmful substances.

This can lead to ineffective treatment or even health risks for those using these supplements. It is important to thoroughly research the brand and source of any medicinal mushroom supplements before making a purchase.

Not suitable for everyone

Pregnant or breastfeeding women, young children, and individuals with certain health conditions should exercise caution before consuming medicinal mushrooms. These fungi contain various bioactive compounds and may interact with certain medications or cause adverse effects in susceptible individuals.

Pregnant or breastfeeding women should avoid them altogether as there is insufficient research on their safety during these periods. Moreover, young children and individuals with compromised immune systems should also consult with their healthcare providers before taking any supplements containing medicinal mushrooms.

Despite these potential disadvantages, most people can safely enjoy the benefits of medicinal mushrooms by choosing high-quality supplements and discussing any concerns with their healthcare provider. Ultimately, the potential benefits of these amazing fungi far outweigh any potential risks or drawbacks.

CHAPTER 3: USE CASES

Medicinal mushrooms are believed to have a wide range of potential health benefits. Some health problems that may be treated or alleviated by using medicinal mushrooms include:

Immune system disorders

Both reishi and maitake mushrooms have been found to contain beta-glucans, polysaccharides that have been shown to stimulate immune system response. Studies have suggested that these compounds can help regulate the immune system, potentially leading to benefits for individuals with autoimmune conditions such as rheumatoid arthritis or lupus.

Additionally, some research has suggested that the antioxidant properties of these medicinal mushrooms may provide further support for immune system health. While more research is needed, these findings suggest that incorporating these mushrooms into one's diet may be a beneficial approach for those with immune system disorders.

Inflammation-related conditions

Cordyceps and Lion's Mane are two medicinal mushrooms that have been identified as having potent anti-inflammatory properties. These mushrooms have been used traditionally to support immunity and manage inflammatory conditions such as arthritis and allergies.

Studies have shown that they contain compounds that reduce inflammation by inhibiting the activity of pro-inflammatory cytokines, thereby alleviating symptoms associated with these conditions. Cordyceps and Lion's Mane have been considered promising alternatives for addressing inflammation-related ailments, with no adverse side effects.

Cardiovascular disease

Medicinal mushrooms have been found to offer promising potential in preventing or managing heart disease. Their cholesterol-lowering and blood pressure-lowering effects have been attributed to bioactive compounds such as beta-glucans, ergothioneine, and phenols.

Additionally, the compounds present in medicinal mushrooms may have anti-inflammatory properties that reduce the risk of atherosclerosis, a condition characterized by the hardening and narrowing of arteries caused by plaque buildup. Overall, medicinal mushrooms offer a natural and potentially effective approach to cardiovascular disease prevention and management.

High cholesterol

Shiitake and oyster mushrooms have unique compounds that can help reduce cholesterol levels. These medicinal mushrooms contain beta-glucans, a type of soluble fiber that binds to cholesterol in the gut, preventing its absorption into the bloodstream. Additionally, they are rich in ergosterol, a precursor to vitamin D that can help regulate cholesterol synthesis in the liver.

Clinical studies have shown that regular consumption of these mushrooms can lower LDL (or "bad") cholesterol levels by up to 30%. These findings make them attractive as a natural alternative to traditional cholesterol-lowering medications.

Diabetes

Shiitake and maitake mushrooms contain bioactive compounds that may help regulate blood sugar levels, making them promising natural remedies for managing diabetes. These mushrooms have been found to increase insulin sensitivity, decrease insulin resistance, and improve glucose metabolism.

They also possess anti-inflammatory properties that can alleviate the chronic low-grade inflammation present in diabetes. Moreover, several studies have reported decreased levels of HbA1C, a marker of long-term blood sugar control, in diabetic patients who consumed shiitake and maitake extracts. Hence, incorporating these medicinal mushrooms into the diet may be beneficial for individuals with diabetes.

Fatigue and stress

Medicinal mushrooms have been found to provide numerous benefits to the human body, especially in terms of stress and fatigue management. Various species contain adaptogenic compounds that can regulate the body's response to stress and reduce the symptoms of fatigue.

In addition, these mushrooms can also help boost immune function, enhance cognitive performance, and regulate mood. The adaptogens present in medicinal mushrooms work by modulating the hypothalamic-pituitary-adrenal (HPA) axis, which is the body's primary stress response system.

Accordingly, consuming these mushrooms may promote a sense of calmness, focus, and well-being. Overall, the health advantages of consuming medicinal mushrooms, particularly for stress and fatigue relief, cannot be underestimated in our fast-paced society.

Digestive issues

Turkey Tail and Chaga are two medicinal mushrooms that have been shown to aid in digestive health. Studies have demonstrated that both mushrooms have prebiotic effects, meaning they promote the growth and activity of beneficial gut bacteria.

Turkey tail has been found to reduce inflammation in the digestive tract and alleviate symptoms of irritable bowel syndrome, while Chaga has been shown to improve digestion and reduce gastrointestinal irritation. These mushrooms may be a promising natural alternative for those suffering from digestive issues.

Skin conditions

Medical experts and researchers are optimistic about the significant potential of mushroom extracts in alleviating a variety of skin conditions. These extracts are believed to possess anti-inflammatory and antioxidant properties that can benefit skin health.

Preliminary studies have indicated that certain medicinal mushroom compounds can help reduce inflammation, prevent oxidative damage, and improve skin texture and hydration. While further research is needed, these findings suggest that mushroom extracts may become an effective, safe, and natural option for addressing skin issues.

Mental health conditions

The neuroprotective effects of compounds found in medicinal mushrooms, such as lion's mane, have been a focus of research in the potential treatment of mental health conditions. Recent studies suggest that these compounds may improve cognitive function, reduce symptoms of anxiety, and alleviate depression.

This is attributed to the ability of these compounds to stimulate the growth of nerve cells and enhance the production of nerve growth factors, which are essential for brain health and function. Further research is needed to confirm these findings.

By incorporating medicinal mushrooms into their diet or supplement regimen, individuals may be able to experience these potential benefits and support their overall health and well-being. However, it's important to discuss any changes to your supplement regimen with a healthcare provider to ensure safety and efficacy.

CHAPTER 4: A 5-STEP GUIDE ON HOW TO GET STARTED WITH MEDICINAL MUSHROOMS

For those new to the world of medicinal mushrooms, getting started can seem daunting. However, with a few simple steps, anyone can incorporate these amazing fungi into their daily routine. Here's a beginner's 5-step guide on how to get started with medicinal mushrooms:

- **Step-1: Do your research**

Each type of medicinal mushroom possesses its own special set of qualities and advantages. For example, reishi is renowned for its relaxing effects, whereas chaga is thought to have characteristics that strengthen the immune system. It is believed that cordyceps can aid increase athletic performance, while lion's mane improves cognitive function.

Spend some time learning about the various kinds of medicinal mushrooms and the possible benefits associated with each of them so that you may evaluate which ones, based on your requirements, have the best chance of helping you.

- **Step-2: Find a reputable supplier**

When looking to purchase medicinal mushrooms, it is essential to locate a seller who has a solid reputation and can be relied upon. Look for businesses that can provide medicinal mushrooms and have a solid reputation in the sector where you intend to sell them.

You can also check to see if the product has been certified by a third party and if it has been tested in a laboratory to confirm its quality and purity. This is of utmost significance because there is a possibility that certain types of mushrooms contain dangerous chemicals or heavy metals.

- **Step-3: Choose your form**

Powders, capsules, extracts, and teas are just some of the many forms that medicinal mushrooms can be found in. Take into account your lifestyle and personal preferences when deciding which method will provide you with the best results while also being the most convenient. For instance, if you are constantly on the move, capsules or extract powders may be more convenient for you, whereas if you enjoy sipping on something warm, tea may be the ideal option for you.

- **Step-4: Start with a low dose**

It is best practice to begin taking a new dietary supplement or herbal medicine in a modest dose whenever possible. This gives you the ability to monitor how your body responds and alter the dosage accordingly. Always make sure to take the product according to the instructions on the label, and only gradually increase the dosage if necessary.

It is important to be aware that certain mushrooms may mix with specific medications or have negative effects in excessive dosages; as a result, it is always preferable to see a healthcare provider prior to using any new supplement.

- **Step-5: Be patient**

Mushrooms used for medicinal purposes operate in a manner distinct from that of medicines and may require more time to manifest their benefits. To get all of the benefits of your use of this product, it is critical to exercise patience and be consistent.

It's possible that seeing the finest outcomes will also depend on whether or not you include medicinal mushrooms in your regular regimen. Remember that the outcomes may vary from person to person and that it may take several weeks or even months before you see any meaningful changes.

By following these simple steps, anyone can get started with medicinal mushrooms and begin reaping the potential health benefits they offer. As always, it's important to discuss any changes to your supplement regimen with a healthcare provider to ensure safety and efficacy.

Safety Considerations

While medicinal mushrooms are generally safe, there are a few safety considerations to keep in mind:

- **Allergies**

It is crucial to exercise caution when consuming medicinal mushrooms due to potential allergies. Those who are new to trying out mushrooms are advised to start with a small dose, especially if they have never tried a specific type of mushroom before. This is because different mushrooms can contain varying compounds that may trigger an allergic reaction in some individuals.

In addition, it is also important to source mushrooms from reputable growers to ensure their safety and potency. As with any other natural supplement or medication, it is recommended to consult with a healthcare professional before incorporating medicinal mushrooms into one's health routine.

- **Interactions with medication**

It's crucial to prioritize safety when incorporating medicinal mushrooms into one's health regimen. While they can provide a range of benefits, it's important to acknowledge the potential for interactions with certain medications.

Consulting with a healthcare provider beforehand can ensure that potential risks are minimized and assist in achieving the best possible health outcomes. Patients should be open and transparent about all medications and supplements they are taking to facilitate the most accurate and informed consultation.

- **Quality control**

Choosing a reputable brand for medicinal mushroom supplements is important to ensure the product's potency and efficacy. The supplement's quality can vary depending on factors such as the extraction method, manufacturing process, and species of mushroom used. By selecting brands that use standardized extracts, have been third-party tested, and follow good manufacturing practices, consumers can ensure they are getting a safe and effective product.

- **Toxicity**

While medicinal mushrooms are generally considered safe for consumption, some species can be toxic. It's important to only consume mushrooms that have been properly identified and are known to be safe for consumption. Mushrooms should be purchased from reputable sources, and any wild mushrooms should be identified by an expert mycologist before being consumed to avoid potential toxicity.

- **Dosage**

It is essential to be cautious when taking these supplements and follow the recommended dosages. Consuming a higher dosage may result in adverse effects such as nausea, diarrhea, and stomach upset. Hence, it is advisable to begin with a low dose when trying a new mushroom for the first time.

Besides, it's worth noting that everyone's tolerance level may differ; therefore, it's critical to monitor your body's response to the supplement. Taking the appropriate dosage is crucial to avoid any unnecessary health risks.

- **Pregnancy and breastfeeding**

The safety of medicinal mushrooms during pregnancy and breastfeeding is not yet fully understood due to limited research. Therefore, it's best to exercise caution and avoid using them unless recommended by a healthcare provider.

Pregnant or breastfeeding women should consult with a healthcare professional before adding any new supplements to their routine to ensure the safety of both themselves and their babies.

- **Autoimmune diseases**

When it comes to using medicinal mushrooms for immune system stimulation, it's crucial to consider the potential safety risks, particularly for individuals with autoimmune diseases such as rheumatoid arthritis and lupus. While beneficial for some conditions, medicinal mushrooms may exacerbate autoimmune symptoms and should be approached with caution.

Consulting with a healthcare provider is highly recommended to ensure the safe and appropriate usage of medicinal mushrooms. It's important to note that even in healthy individuals, it's crucial to follow recommended dosages and avoid long-term use to prevent adverse effects on the liver, kidneys, and other organs.

- **Surgery**

Medicinal mushrooms have become increasingly popular for their various health benefits. However, it's important to note that these supplements may increase the risk of bleeding during surgery. This is due to their anticoagulant properties, which can interfere with the body's ability to form clots and stop bleeding.

To ensure a safe surgery, patients should stop taking these supplements at least 2 weeks before their scheduled procedure. It's crucial to inform healthcare providers about the use of medicinal mushrooms to prevent potential complications, as well as to follow their instructions for a successful recovery.

- **Children**

When it comes to the safety of medicinal mushrooms for children, it is important to seek advice from a healthcare provider. While they are generally safe for adults, there is little research on their efficacy and potential side effects on children.

Therefore, parents should exercise caution when considering giving these supplements to their little ones. As such, it is always best to consult with a healthcare professional before administering medicinal mushrooms to children to ensure their safety and well-being.

- **Storage and preparation**

Proper storage and preparation of medicinal mushrooms are crucial to reduce the risk of foodborne illness. These mushrooms should be stored in airtight containers in the refrigerator and consumed within a few days of purchase. It's important to wash them thoroughly before cooking and to cook them at a sufficient temperature to kill any harmful bacteria or viruses.

Medicinal mushrooms have numerous health benefits, but consuming them without taking proper safety precautions can lead to serious health issues. Therefore, it's important to handle medicinal mushrooms with care to reap their maximum benefits.

While medicinal mushrooms are generally safe and well-tolerated, it's important to be cautious and follow recommended dosages, choose reputable brands, and consult with a healthcare provider if you have any concerns or questions.

Conclusion

Congratulations! You've made it to the end of our journey exploring the fascinating world of medicinal mushrooms. Hopefully, you've learned a lot about these incredible fungi and have been inspired to try incorporating them into your daily routine.

From boosting your immune system and reducing inflammation to improving your overall mood and cognitive function, medicinal mushrooms offer a wide range of benefits for just about everyone. Whether you're looking to improve your physical health or your mental clarity, there's a mushroom out there that can help you achieve your goals.

One of the best things about medicinal mushrooms is that they're entirely natural, meaning you can feel good about adding them to your diet without worrying about any harmful side effects. Unlike some other supplements or medications, mushrooms won't interfere with other aspects of your life, so you can continue doing everything you love while enjoying their many benefits.

So go ahead and give medicinal mushrooms a try! Incorporate them into your daily routine in whatever way works best for you — whether it's mixing them into your morning coffee or taking a supplement capsule — and see how they can enhance your overall well-being.

But remember, not all mushrooms are created equal, and it's important to do your research before diving in. Make sure you purchase mushrooms from reputable sources that have been sustainably sourced and processed for maximum effectiveness. And as always, consult with your healthcare provider before making any significant changes to your diet or supplement regimen.

In conclusion, medicinal mushrooms are one of nature's most valuable gifts, offering an impressive array of benefits to support your body and mind. By incorporating them into your daily routine, you can take advantage of their many health-boosting properties while enjoying a natural and safe way to improve your overall quality of life.

So why wait? Start exploring the world of medicinal mushrooms today and discover all that these little wonders have to offer. Your body and mind will thank you!

FAQ

1. What are medicinal mushrooms?

Medicinal mushrooms are fungi that have been used for centuries in traditional medicine practices around the world. They contain a variety of beneficial compounds, including beta-glucans, polysaccharides, and triterpenes, which have been shown to support our immune system, reduce inflammation, and improve our overall health and well-being.

2. What are some common types of medicinal mushrooms?

There are many different types of medicinal mushrooms, each with its unique set of properties. Some of the most popular include Reishi, Chaga, Cordyceps, Lion's Mane, and Turkey Tail.

3. How do I consume medicinal mushrooms?

There are many ways to consume medicinal mushrooms, including through supplements, teas, powders, capsules, and tinctures. You can even cook with certain types of mushrooms or add them to your favorite recipes for an added health boost.

4. Are there any side effects of consuming medicinal mushrooms?

While medicinal mushrooms are considered safe for most people, they can have some potential side effects. These may include upset stomach, diarrhea, and allergic reactions. It's always a good idea to check with your healthcare provider before consuming medicinal mushrooms, especially if you have any underlying health conditions or are taking any medications.

5. Can children consume medicinal mushrooms?

Yes, children can consume medicinal mushrooms, but it's important to start with small doses and consult with a healthcare provider first. Certain types of mushrooms, such as Reishi, may be better suited for children due to their milder taste and gentle properties.

6. Can medicinal mushrooms interfere with other medications or supplements?

Certain types of medicinal mushrooms can interact with medications and supplements, so it's always a good idea to check with your healthcare provider before consuming them. For example, Chaga may interact with blood thinners, while Cordyceps may interact with immunosuppressant medications.

7. Where can I purchase high-quality medicinal mushrooms?

There are many places where you can purchase high-quality medicinal mushrooms, including health food stores, online retailers, and specialty shops. It's important to do your research and choose a reputable source that offers sustainably sourced and processed mushrooms for maximum effectiveness.

References and Helpful Links

Venturella, G., Ferraro, V., Cirlincione, F., & Gargano, M. L. (2021). Medicinal Mushrooms: Bioactive Compounds, Use, and Clinical Trials. International Journal of Molecular Sciences, 22(2), 634. https://doi.org/10.3390/ijms22020634

Törős, G., El-Ramady, H., Prokisch, J., Velasco, F., Llanaj, X., Nguyen, D. H. H., & Peles, F. (2023). Modulation of the Gut Microbiota with Prebiotics and Antimicrobial Agents from Pleurotus ostreatus Mushroom. Foods, 12(10), 2010. https://doi.org/10.3390/foods12102010

Amitahc. (2023, February 28). MyCodry: the hidden power of Mushrooms - Amita hc. Amita Hc. https://www.amitahc.com/news/mycodry-the-hidden-power-of-mushrooms/#:~:text=Shiitake%20can%20in%20fact%20po sitively,from%20the%20liver%2C%20protecting%20circulati on.

Zhang, J., & An, J. (2007). Cytokines, Inflammation, and Pain. International Anesthesiology Clinics, 45(2), 27–37. https://doi.org/10.1097/aia.0b013e318034194e

Lovegrove, A., Edwards, C. H., Brasca, M., Patel, H., El, S. N., Grassby, T., Zielke, C. W., Ulmius, M., Nilsson, L., Butterworth, P. J., Ellis, P. R., & Shewry, P. R. (2017). Role of polysaccharides in food, digestion, and health. Critical Reviews in Food Science and Nutrition, 57(2), 237–253. https://doi.org/10.1080/10408398.2014.939263

Mushrooms. (2022, March 2). The Nutrition Source. https://www.hsph.harvard.edu/nutritionsource/food-features/mushrooms/

Park, H. (2022). Current Uses of Mushrooms in Cancer Treatment and Their Anticancer Mechanisms. International Journal of Molecular Sciences, 23(18), 10502. https://doi.org/10.3390/ijms231810502

Mushrooms, R. (2022b). Medicinal Mushrooms: 7 Kinds and Their Unique Health Benefits. Real Mushrooms. https://www.realmushrooms.com/7-medicinal-mushroom-benefits-for-health/